Table of Contents

INTRODUCTION

Diverticulitis is a common gastrointestinal condition that occurs when small pouches (diverticula) in the lining of the digestive tract become inflamed or infected. This can lead to abdominal pain, bloating, changes in bowel habits, and other unpleasant symptoms. Proper dietary management is an essential part of managing diverticulitis and preventing flare-ups.

The diverticulitis diet is designed to provide relief during acute flare-ups and to promote long-term digestive health. **The main goals of the diet are to:**

• **Reduce inflammation:** Certain foods can help calm inflammation in the digestive tract, alleviating the painful symptoms of diverticulitis.

• **Promote regular bowel movements:** Keeping stools soft and regular can help prevent further irritation and complications.

• **Provide adequate nutrition:** The diet ensures you get the necessary nutrients for overall health, even during periods of flare-ups.

During an acute diverticulitis attack, the diet typically recommends a liquid or low-fiber diet to give the digestive system a chance to rest and heal. This may include clear broths, juices, and smooth, non-dairy-based soups. Solid foods are gradually reintroduced as the inflammation subsides.

Once the acute phase has passed, the focus shifts to a high-fiber, plant-based diet to promote regular bowel movements and overall gut health. This includes:

• **Whole grains:** Opt for whole wheat, brown rice, oats, and other whole grain breads, cereals, and pastas.

• **Fruits and vegetables:** Aim for a variety of fresh, canned, or frozen produce, focusing on those with soluble fiber like berries, pears, and broccoli.

• **Legumes:** Beans, lentils, and other legumes are excellent sources of fiber and can be slowly reintroduced into the diet.

• **Nuts and seeds:** These provide healthy fats and fiber, but should be consumed in moderation, as they can be difficult to digest during flare-ups.

It's important to gradually increase your fiber intake, as suddenly consuming large amounts can worsen symptoms. Drinking plenty of water throughout the day is also crucial to keep stools soft and regular.

In addition to the dietary guidelines, the diverticulitis diet also recommends:

1. Limiting red meat and processed meats, which may contribute to inflammation.

2. Avoiding foods that can cause gas or bloating, such as carbonated beverages, cruciferous vegetables, and dairy products (if you're lactose intolerant).

3. Staying hydrated by drinking plenty of water and other non-caffeinated, non-alcoholic beverages.

4. Engaging in regular physical activity, which can help promote healthy digestion.

Diverticulitis is the inflammation of the diverticula — or small pouches — located along your digestive tract.

If you have these pouches, it's called diverticulosis.

These diverticula can become inflamed or infected if they become blocked with stool or partially digested food, which can cause the build-up of bacteria.

This inflammation can cause severe left lower stomach pain, the most common symptom of diverticulitis.

In Asian people, however, the pain is more often located on the right side.

If this pain is severe enough and you develop complications, you may require hospitalization.

Other symptoms of diverticulitis include:

• nausea

• vomiting

• low-grade fever

• diarrhea

• constipation

You may also notice blood in your stools, but the stomach pain associated with diverticulitis does not usually occur with the bleeding.

Several risk factors can contribute to the development of diverticulitis.

These factors include:

• increasing age

• excess body weight

• smoking

• low fiber intake

• high red meat intake

• physical inactivity

Genetic factors and the use of certain medications like nonsteroidal anti-inflammatory drugs (NSAIDs) can also increase the risk of diverticulitis.

Proper nutrition plays a vital role in managing diverticulitis and can also lower the chances of recurrence. Diverticulitis occurs when small pouches along the digestive tract, especially in the large intestine, become inflamed or infected.

Though these pouches are typically harmless, they can lead to diverticulitis when inflamed. Managing diverticulitis symptoms involves adopting specific dietary choices while avoiding others. This resource outlines dietary recommendations for both diverticulitis and diverticulosis, offering a three-day sample menu with recipes suitable for home preparation and enjoyment with family and friends.

DIVERTICULITIS DIET

The diet recommendations for diverticulitis depend on its severity.

If you're experiencing diverticulitis with complications, your doctor may restrict you from consuming food or beverages by mouth (NPO).

This provides your bowels with rest until you're medically stable.

If you have no complications, your doctor will likely start you on clear liquids for hydration and then advance your diet to a low-fiber or bland diet until you start to feel better.

A clear liquid diet consists exclusively of translucent liquids such as tea, coffee, clear soda, broths, and some nutrition supplements like Ensure Clear.

However, you may wish to avoid caffeinated beverages as they may worsen your symptoms.

A low-fiber diet can reduce the frequency and volume of your stools, helping to reduce inflammation of your large intestine so that it can heal.

It's recommended to follow a low-fiber diet — which restricts fiber to 10 grams per day — until you start to feel better, which may take two to three days.

Additionally, you should include protein with each meal to promote intestinal healing.

Foods to avoid

Limit high-fiber and high-fat foods that can slow digestion.

Examples of foods to avoid with diverticulitis include:

• **Grains:** cereals, popcorn, oatmeal, brown rice, and whole-grain bread, pasta, and tortillas

• **Seeds and nuts:** almonds, Brazil nuts, chia seeds, flaxseed, sunflower seeds, walnuts, etc.

• **Legumes:** beans, peas, and lentils

• **Protein:** fried meat and processed meats, such as bologna, salami, sausage, bacon, and hot dogs

• **Dairy:** whole milk, cream, sour cream, and yogurt with added fruit, nuts, and granola

• **Vegetables:** raw or undercooked vegetables, including beets, broccoli, corn, cucumbers, peas, potato skins, spinach, and tomatoes

• **Fruits:** raw or dried fruit, canned fruit with mandarin oranges or pineapple, prune juice, and fruit skin

Avoiding alcohol is also helpful during a diverticulitis flare-up as it may worsen your symptoms.

The caffeine from coffee and tea can also worsen symptoms in some people.

Foods to eat

Consume low-fiber foods that are easy to digest.

These foods include:

• **Grains:** cream of wheat, white rice, enriched white bread, crackers, pasta, white flour, corn tortillas

• **Protein:** fish, pork, chicken, eggs, tofu

• **Dairy:** low-fat milk, cheddar or parmesan cheese, cottage cheese, and yogurt without nuts, fruit, or granola

• **Vegetables:** cooked carrots or green beans, potatoes without skin, strained vegetable juice

• **Fruits:** fruit juice, canned peaches, pears, applesauce, very ripe bananas

3-day sample diverticulitis diet menu

Here is a three-day sample diverticulitis diet menu that is low in fiber and provides protein with each meal:

Day 1

- Breakfast: cream of wheat and scrambled eggs

- Lunch: tuna sandwich on white bread

- Snack: whey protein supplement and very ripe banana (2 grams of fiber)

- Dinner: pork chop, white rice, and cooked carrots

Day 2 (vegan)

- Breakfast: tofu scramble and white toast

- Lunch: vegan tomato basil soup with French baguette

- Snack: vegan protein powder and very ripe banana

- Dinner: sweet potato quinoa salad without beans

Day 3

- Breakfast: puff cereal and canned pears

- Lunch: chicken noodle soup

- Snack: low-fat cottage cheese with canned peaches

- Dinner: chicken breast, white rice, and canned green beans

How to reduce diverticulitis flare-ups

It is estimated that 20–50% of individuals will experience recurrent episodes of diverticulitis.

However, adopting a high-fiber diet and maintaining an active lifestyle can significantly lower this risk and mitigate potential complications associated with future episodes of diverticulitis.

High-fiber diet for diverticulitis

While a diet low in fiber may be beneficial during recuperation from diverticulitis, transitioning to a high-fiber diet post-recovery can aid in averting future occurrences. Studies also indicate that adhering to a high-fiber diet can decrease the likelihood of hospitalization stemming from diverticulitis.

The best sources of fiber include:

- fruits, all types, especially those with skins

- vegetables, especially raw

• whole grains, including popcorn, oatmeal, brown rice, and whole-wheat bread

• nuts and seeds

• legumes, such as beans, peas, and lentils

Historically, the belief was that nuts, seeds, and popcorn should be avoided due to concerns about them potentially causing diverticulitis by getting stuck in the diverticula.

However, there's no evidence to support this claim. Instead, these foods should be consumed for their fiber content. For example, a study involving over 50,000 women found that a higher intake of fiber from fruits and whole grains was associated with a reduced risk of diverticulitis.

Specifically, the risk decreased by 5% for every serving of fruit consumed by the women. Similarly, another study with more than 46,000 men yielded similar results, showing that a fiber-rich diet was linked to a decreased risk of diverticulitis.

Conversely, the same study found that the Western pattern diet, high in red meat, refined grains, and added sugars, was associated with an increased risk of diverticulitis. While these foods don't directly trigger diverticulitis, excessive consumption of them, especially without enough fiber from fruits, vegetables, and whole grains, can elevate your risk.

A high-fiber diet can help reduce the risk of diverticulitis by increasing stool bulk and decreasing pressure on your large intestine.

Fiber also promotes the growth of beneficial bacteria in your gut, which reduces inflammation and supports intestinal health. Aim to consume 25–35 grams of fiber per day and ensure you stay hydrated. If you're not currently following a high-fiber diet, gradually increase your fiber intake to avoid stomach discomfort and constipation.

Vigorous exercise

Like a high-fiber diet, exercise has also been associated with a reduced risk of diverticulitis or hospitalization due to the condition.

For example, an observational study of more than 47,000 men found that those who engaged in vigorous physical activity were less likely to experience diverticulitis and bleeding than those who engaged in moderately intense physical activity.

Based on this study, the American Gastroenterological Association Institute guidelines recommend regular vigorous physical activity to reduce the risk of diverticulitis.

The Physical Activity Guidelines for Americans recommend 75–150 minutes per week of vigorous-intensity exercise.

Here are some examples of vigorous-intensity exercise:

• jogging

- running

- bicycling

- swimming

- playing basketball

- playing soccer

Vigorous exercise may decrease the risk of diverticulitis due to its positive effects on the gastrointestinal tract and by reducing inflammation.

Still, while vigorous physical activity may offer the greatest benefits, exercise or activity of any intensity can be beneficial.

DIVERTICULITIS DIET CUISINE COOKBOOK

BREAKFAST

Multigrain Pancakes

Ingredients

- 1 1/2 Cup plain yogurt

- 1/2 Cup milk

- 2 eggs

- 3 Tablespoons canola oil

- 1 Cup whole wheat flour

* 1/3 Cup flour

* 1/3 Cup quick cooking oats

* 2 Teaspoons baking powder

* 1/2 Teaspoon baking soda

* Non-stick cooking spray

Instructions

* In a medium bowl, combine yogurt, milk, eggs, and oil. Mix well.

* In a separate bowl, combine flours, oats, baking powder and soda. Mix well. Add dry ingredients to wet ingredients and mix just to moisten.

* Spray a non-stick pan with non-stick cooking spray and heat pan over medium heat. For each pancake, pour slightly less than 1/4 cup batter from cup into hot pan.

* Cook pancakes until puffed and dry around edges. Turn and cook other side until golden. Serve pancakes with warm maple syrup and fruit if desired.

Oatmeal Pumpkin Raisin Pancakes
Ingredients

* 1 1/2 Cup rolled oats

- 1/2 Cup whole wheat flour

- 1 Tablespoon baking powder

- 1 Teaspoon cinnamon

- 1 Teaspoon nutmeg

- egg

- banana, mashed

- 1 Tablespoon honey

- 1/2 Cup pumpkin puree, canned

- 1 1/2 Cup milk

- 1/2 Cup seedless raisins

- Non-stick cooking spray

Instructions

- In a large bowl mix together oats, whole wheat flour, baking powder, cinnamon, and nutmeg. Set aside.

- In a separate bowl, mix together egg, banana, honey, pumpkin puree, milk and raisins or dates. Mix dry mixture into wet mixture.

- Heat griddle or skillet over medium heat. Spray with non-stick cooking spray.

19

• For each pancake, pour slightly less than 1/4 cup batter from cup into hot griddle or pan. Cook pancakes until puffed and dry around edges. Turn and cook other side until golden.

Pumpkin Pie Oatmeal

Ingredients

• 1/2 Cup rolled oats

• 3/4 Cups milk or water

• 1/2 Cup pumpkin puree

• 1 Teaspoon brown sugar

• 1 Teaspoon pumpkin spice

Instructions

• In a microwave-safe bowl, mix together oats, milk or water and pumpkin puree.

• Cook in microwave on high for 45 seconds. Stir and microwave for another 30 seconds.

• Sprinkle with brown sugar and pumpkin spice and add a splash of milk.

Sante Fe Omelet

Ingredients

- 4 eggs

- 2 Tablespoons milk or water

- 1/4 Teaspoon salt

- 1 1/2 Tablespoon butter

- 1/2 Cup red beans, drained, rinsed

- tomato, seeded, chopped

- 1/2 Cup green bell pepper, seeded, chopped

- Tablespoons cheddar cheese, grated

- Pieces whole wheat tortillas

Instructions

- In a medium bowl, whisk together eggs, milk or water and salt.

- Heat butter in a medium skillet and add red beans. Cook for 3 minutes, add tomatoes and green peppers.

- Cook for another 5 minutes until vegetables soften. Pour in egg mixture and sprinkle the cheese over the eggs.

- Cover until cheese melts. Serve with whole wheat tortillas.

Apple and Pear Pita Pockets

Ingredients

- 1/2 small apple, unpeeled, chopped

- 1/2 small pear, unpeeled, chopped

- 1/4 Cup cottage cheese

- 1 whole wheat pita bread

Instructions

- Combine the apple, pear, and cottage cheese in a bowl.

- Slice the pita bread to make a pocket. Fill the pocket with the fruit mixture.

- Sprinkle some cinnamon or drizzle a little honey or agave syrup for added sweetness.

Apple Raisin Pancakes

Ingredients

- 2 eggs

- 1 Cup unsweetened applesauce

- 1 Teaspoon cinnamon

- 2 Teaspoons brown sugar

- 1 Cup wheat flour

- 1/2 Cup white flour

- 2 Teaspoons baking powder

- 2 Teaspoons vanilla

- 1/2 Cup golden, seedless raisins

- non-stick cooking spray

Instructions

- In a medium bowl, beat eggs until fluffy.

- Add applesauce, cinnamon, sugar, flours, baking powder, vanilla and raisins and continue to stir just until smooth.

- Heat griddle or pan over medium heat. Spray with non-stick cooking spray. For each pancake, pour about 1/4 cup of batter into hot pan.

- Cook pancakes until edges get puffy. Turn and cook other side unti golden. Serve pancakes with additional applesauce if desired.

Apricot Honey Oatmeal

Ingredients

23

- 1 Cup water or milk or almond milk

- 1/4 Cup dried apricots, chopped

- 1/2 Cup rolled oats

- 1 Tablespoon honey

- 1/4 Teaspoon cinnamon

Instructions

- Place water or milk, apricots, honey, and cinnamon and oats in a microwave-safe bowl.

- Cook in microwave for about 2 minutes until most of the liquid is absorbed, stirring occasionally.

Asparagus and Bean Frittata

Ingredients

- 2 Tablespoons olive oil

- 1 Cup onion, chopped

- 1 Cup red pepper, seeded, chopped

- garlic clove, minced

- 14 Ounces can red or black or white beans, drained, rinsed

- 1 Cup asparagus, cooked and chopped

- 4 eggs

- 1/2 Teaspoon salt

- 1/4 Cup Parmesan cheese

Instructions

- Preheat oven to 350 degrees.

- In a large oven-proof pan, heat 1 tbsp olive oil over medium-high heat. Cook onions, red peppers, garlic, and red beans until vegetables are soft (about 10 minutes). Set aside.

- In medium bowl, beat eggs and salt, then add asparagus; set aside.

- Add remaining 1 tbsp olive oil into the vegetable pan and pour in the egg mixture. Reduce heat to medium-low and cook for 10 to 15 minutes, or until mixture is set on bottom and lightly browned.

- Sprinkle Parmesan cheese over top of mixture and broil in the oven for an additional 3 to 5 minutes or until cheese is lightly browned and eggs are cooked through.

Banana Bran Muffins

Ingredients

- 1 ½ Cup All-Bran cereal

- 2/3 Cups milk

- 4 eggs

- 1/4 Cup canola oil

- 1 Cup ripe banana, mashed (about 2 bananas)

- 1/2 Cup brown sugar

- 1 Cup whole wheat flour

- 2 Teaspoons baking powder

- 1/2 Teaspoon salt

Instructions

- Preheat oven to 400F degrees.

- In a large bowl, combine All-Bran cereal and milk and set aside. Add eggs and oil; stir in mashed banana and brown sugar and combine well.

- In a separate small bowl, combine flour, baking powder and salt. Add dry ingredients to banana mixture, stirring just until combined.

- Pour batter evenly into 12 greased or paper-lined muffin tins; Bake 15 to 18 minutes or until golden-brown and firm. Allow to cool prior to serving.

Banana Breakfast Smoothie

Ingredients

- 1 medium banana

- 1 Cup milk, almond or regular

- 1/2 Cup plain yogurt

- 1/4 Cup 100% Bran flakes

- 1 Teaspoon vanilla extract

- 2 Teaspoons honey or agave syrup

- 1/2 Cup ice

- 1 Pinch cinnamon

- 1 Pinch nutmeg

Instructions

- Combine all ingredients in a blender and process on medium speed until smooth.

- Garnish with cinnamon and/or nutmeg.

Bran Muffins

Ingredients

- 2 Cups All-Bran cereal

- 1/4 Cup brown sugar

- 1/2 Cup butter

- 2 eggs

- 2 Cups buttermilk

- 2 ½ Cups whole wheat flour

- 2 ½ Teaspoons baking soda

- ½ Teaspoon salt

- 1 Cup dates

- 1 Cup seedless raisins

Instructions

- Preheat oven to 400F degrees.

- Soak 1 cup of All-Bran cereal in 1 cup boiling water and set aside. In a mixer, cream sugar and butter together until well blended. Add eggs, one at a time and beat until fluffy. Add buttermilk and soaked bran mixture.

- In a separate bowl, combine flour, baking soda, and salt . Add flour mixture into the batter but do not over mix. Add in remaining 1 cup of cereal, dates and raisins. Pour batter evenly into 10 greased or paper-lined muffin tins.

- Bake 15-20 minutes. Allow to cool prior to serving.

• Soak 1 cup of All-Bran cereal in 1 cup boiling water and set aside.

• In a mixer, cream sugar and butter together until well blended. Add eggs, one at a time and beat until fluffy. Add buttermilk and soaked bran mixture.

• In a separate bowl, combine flour, baking soda, and salt . Add flour mixture into the batter but do not over mix. Add in remaining 1 cup of cereal, dates and raisins.

• Pour batter evenly into 10 greased or paper-lined muffin tins. Bake 15-20 minutes. Allow to cool prior to serving.

Breakfast Carrot Cake

Ingredients

• 1 1/3 Cup water

• 1/2 Cup brown sugar

• 1 Cup seedless raisins

• 2 carrots, grated

• apple, unpeeled, chopped

• 1 Teaspoon cinnamon

• 1 Teaspoon ground cloves

• 1 Teaspoon nutmeg

• Teaspoons butter

* Cups whole wheat flour

* 1 Teaspoon baking soda

Instructions

* Preheat oven to 375F degrees. Spray a 9x5 inch loaf pan with non-stick cooking spray.

* In a medium saucepan, over low heat, mix together water, sugar, raisins, carrots, apples, cinnamon, cloves, nutmeg, and butter. Cook for 5-7 minutes, until well combined, and sugar dissolves. Remove pan from heat and allow to cool.

* In a large bowl, combine flour, baking soda and salt. Stir carrot mixture into flour mixture and mix just until combined.

* Pour into prepared pan. Bake for 1 1/4 hours, or until a knife inserted in the center comes out clean. Cool on wire rack.

Broccoli Omelet

Ingredients

* 8 eggs

* 4 Tablespoons milk

* 1/2 Teaspoon salt

* 1 1/2 Tablespoon extra virgin olive oil

* 1/2 onion, chopped

* 1 Cup broccoli, fresh or frozen and thawed

* 1/2 Cup Monterrey Jack cheese, shredded

Instructions

* In a bowl, whisk together eggs, milk and salt.

* Heat olive oil in a medium skillet over medium-high heat, add onion and broccoli and cook until tender, about 7 minutes. Add the egg mixture, stirring to cook eggs evenly.

* Sprinkle with cheese. Lower heat and cover until cheese melts. Flip over in half and serve.

Carrot and Zucchini Bread

Ingredients

* 3 1/2 Cups whole wheat flour

* 1 Tablespoon baking powder

* 1 Teaspoon baking soda

* 1/2 Teaspoon salt

* 1 Teaspoon cinnamon

* 2 eggs, lightly beaten

- 1 1/2 Cup buttermilk

- 2 Tablespoons butter, melted

- 1/2 Cup brown sugar

- 1 Cup zucchini, unpeeled, grated

- 1 Cup carrot, grated

- 1 Cup apple, unseeded, grated

Instructions

- Preheat oven to 350F degrees.

- Spray two 9x5-inch loaf pans with non-stick cooking spray. In a bowl, combine the flour, baking powder, baking soda, salt, and cinnamon; set aside.

- In a large, separate bowl, combine the eggs, buttermilk, and melted butter. Stir in the brown sugar. Add the zucchini, carrots, and apple and combine.

- Stir in the dry ingredients into the wet ingredients and stir gently until just combined.

- Pour batter into prepared loaf pans. Bake for 60 minutes, or until a knife inserted into the center of the loaf comes out clean. Cool loaves in the pan for 10 minutes before removing to a wire rack to cool completely.

Sunrise Burrito Wrap

Ingredients

• 1 Tablespoon olive oil

• 2 Slices turkey

• 1/4 Cup green bell pepper, seeded, chopped

• 1/4 Cup black beans

• 2 eggs

• 2 Tablespoons milk

• 1/4 Teaspoon salt

• 2 Tablespoons Monterrey Jack cheese, grated

• whole wheat tortilla

Instructions

• In a small non-stick pan, heat olive oil on medium heat and cook turkey about 2 minutes until slightly crispy.

• Add bell peppers and beans and continue to cook until warmed through.

• In a small bowl beat together egg with milk and salt. Add beaten eggs and stir gently until eggs are almost cooked through.

• Add grated cheese and lower heat to lowest setting. Cover and continue to cook until cheese has completely melted. Place mixture on wheat tortilla and roll into a burrito.

Tropical Fruit Smoothie

Ingredients

- 1 Cup mix of mangoes, pineapples, bananas

- 1 Cup plain or vanilla yogurt

- 1/2 Cup All Bran cereal

- 1 Teaspoon vanilla

- 1 Tablespoon honey, or agave nectar, optional

- 1 Cup almond or coconut milk or water

- 1/2 avocado

- 1 Cup ice

Instructions

• Combine all ingredients in a blender and process on high speed until smooth and creamy.

Zucchini and Bean Scramble

Ingredients

- 2 Tablespoons olive oil

- 1/2 Cup red onions, chopped finely

- medium zucchini, seeded, chopped

- 14 Ounces can black beans, drained, rinsed

- 1/2 tomato, seeded, chopped

- 4 eggs

- 1/4 Cup milk

- 1 Teaspoon salt

- 4 whole wheat English muffins

Instructions

- In a large non-stick pan, heat olive oil over moderate heat.

- Add onions, zucchini, black beans and tomato. Cook for 5-10 minutes or until vegetables are soft.

- In a separate bowl, mix together eggs and milk and salt. Add egg mixture to pan and stir to cook through, about 5 minutes.

- Serve with whole wheat English muffins.

MAIN DISHES

Ingredients

- 1 Pound whole wheat pasta

- 1 Tablespoon olive oil

- 1 onion

- 1 garlic cloves, minced

- 1 Pound ground turkey

- 1 small head escarole, rinsed, drained, and chopped

- 14 Ounces can,cannellini beans, drained and rinsed

- 1 1/2 Cup chicken broth

- 1 Tablespoon fresh rosemary, chopped

- 1/2 Teaspoon salt

- 1/2 Teaspoon pepper

- 1/2 Cup Parmesan cheese

Instructions

- Bring a large pot of salted water to boil. Add pasta and cook according to package directions. Drain.

• In a large pan, heat olive oil over medium heat. Add onion and cook until softened, add garlic and turkey and cook until it browns, about 5-7 minutes.

• Add the escarole and cook until wilted, about 3 to 4 minutes. Add the beans, 1 cup of chicken stock, rosemary, and salt and pepper. Simmer until the mixture is slightly thickened.

• Add the turkey-bean mixture to pasta and toss well, thinning sauce with the additional 1/2 cup chicken stock if necessary.

• Top with parmesan cheese. Serve.

Pasta with Chicken and Olives

Ingredients

• 1 Pound whole wheat pasta

• 2 Tablespoons olive oil

• onion, chopped

• garlic cloves, minced

• 1 Pound chicken breast, cut into chunks

• 1 Teaspoon dried basil

• 1 Teaspoon dried rosemary

• black olives, sliced

• green bell pepper, seeded, chopped

• 14 Ounces can stewed tomatoes, chopped

• 2 Cups chicken broth

• 1/2 Cup Romano cheese

Instructions

• Bring a large pot of salted water to boil. Add pasta and cook according to package directions until al dente.

• While pasta is cooking, heat the oil in a large pan over medium heat. Add the onion and garlic and cook until the onion is tender, about 6 minutes.

• Add the chicken, basil and rosemary and cook until the chicken is lightly browned, about 8 minutes. Stir in the olives, green pepper and tomatoes and cook until the tomatoes begin to give off liquid, about 2 minutes.

• Add the chicken broth to the pan, heat pan to boiling and boil until half of the liquid is evaporated, about 5-7 minutes.

• When pasta is done, add to sauce mixture. Toss until pasta is evenly mixed with sauce. Top with cheese and serve.

Pasta with Spinach and White Beans
Ingredients

- 1 Pound whole wheat pasta

- 2 Tablespoons olive oil

- garlic cloves, minced

- 3 Cups tomatoes, seeded and chopped

- 14 Ounces can,cannellini beans, drained and rinsed

- 1 Cup tomato sauce

- 2 Cups fresh spinach, washed and chopped

- 1/2 Cup Feta cheese, crumbled

Instructions

- Bring a large pot of water to a boil. Add salt and add pasta and cook according to package instructions. Drain.

- In a large pan, heat olive oil over medium heat. Cook garlic for 3 - 4 minutes. Add tomatoes, beans and tomato sauce. Bring to a boil. Reduce heat, cover and let simmer for 20 minutes.

- Add spinach to the sauce and let simmer for another 5 minutes or until spinach wilts. Place cooked pasta in a large serving bowl, pour sauce over pasta and sprinkle feta cheese. Toss to combine. Serve.

Quick Broccoli Pasta Toss

Ingredients

• 2 Cups broccoli florets, fresh or thawed if frozen

• 1/2 p Pound whole wheat pasta

• 1/2 Tablespoon olive oil

• 1 1/2 Tablespoon Parmesan cheese

• 1/8 Teaspoon garlic powder

Instructions

• Bring a large pot of salted water to a boil.

• Add broccoli and pasta and cook for about 6 - 8 minutes or until tender. Drain well.

• Place pasta mixture in a large shallow pasta bowl and toss with olive oil, cheese and garlic powder. Serve.

Red Beans and Rice

Ingredients

• 1 Tablespoon olive oil

• onion, chopped

• stalks celery, chopped

• garlic cloves, minced

- 14 Ounces tomato sauce

- 1/2 Teaspoon oregano

- 1/2 Tablespoon thyme

- 14 Ounces beef stock

- 28 Ounces red beans, drained and rinsed

- 4 Cups cooked brown rice

Instructions

- In a large non-stick pan, heat olive oil over medium heat. Cook onions, celery and garlic stirring until just tender.

- Stir in tomato paste, oregano and thyme. Add beef broth, stir and bring to a boil. Simmer uncovered about 35 minutes or until mixture thickens. Add red beans and let cook until heated through.

- Serve over brown rice.

Rice and Vegetable Casserole

Ingredients

- Non-stick cooking spray

- 1 Cup long-grain brown rice

- 1/4 Cup mushrooms, sliced

- 1/4 Cup broccoli, chopped

- 1/4 Cup carrots, chopped

- 1/4 Cup red bell pepper, seeded and chopped

- 1/4 Cup onion, finely chopped

- 1 Teaspoon salt

- 1 Teaspoon paprika

- 1 Teaspoon oregano

- 2-2 1/2 Cups vegetable broth

- 1/4 Cup cheddar cheese, shredded

Instructions

- Preheat oven to 425 degrees. Spray a 13x9 glass baking dish lightly with non-stick cooking spray.

- In a large bowl, combine brown rice, mushrooms, broccoli, carrots, bell pepper, onion, salt, paprika, oregano, and broth. Mix well until all ingredients are incorporated. Transfer the mixture into the greased 13x9 baking dish and cover with foil.

- Bake casserole dish in preheated oven for 30 minutes, or until cooked through; stir once half way during baking.

- Top with shredded cheddar cheese and allow it to melt prior to serving.

Ingredients

- 1 Cup long-grain brown rice

- 1/4 Cup soy sauce, low sodium preferred

- 2 Tablespoons rice vinegar

- 1/4 Cup lemon juice

- 2 Tablespoons honey

- 1 Tablespoon olive oil

- 1 Pound medium shrimp, cleaned, peeled and deveined

- 8 Ounces snow peas, cut in halves

- ginger piece, 1 inch long, shredded

- avocado, sliced

Instructions

- In a large saucepan, bring 2 cups of water to a boil. Add the rice and cover and reduce heat to simmer. Cook until rice is tender and water has evaporated, about 35-45 minutes.

- While rice is cooking, in a small bowl, combine soy sauce, lemon juice, vinegar, and honey until well combined and set aside.

• In a large non-stick pan, heat olive oil over medium-high heat. Cook shrimp with peas and ginger until shrimp turn pink, about 3-4 minutes.

• To serve, place rice on plate and top with shrimp mixture and chopped avocado. Serve the sauce on the side.

Roasted Chicken and Vegetables

Ingredients

• Roma tomatoes, seedless, quartered

• zucchini, medium, chopped coarsely

• potatoes, large, unpeeled, quartered

• 3 Tablespoons olive oil, divided

• 3/4 Teaspoons salt, divided

• garlic cloves, minced

• 1 Tablespoon fresh rosemary, chopped

• 1 Tablespoon fresh thyme, taken off sprig

• 1 Teaspoon lemon zest

• 1 Tablespoon lemon juice

• chicken breast halves, skinless

Instructions

• Preheat oven to 375F degrees.

• Place tomatoes, zucchini and potatoes in a large roasting pan, and toss with 2 tbs of oil and 1/4 tsp salt.

• In a small bowl, combine 1 tbs oil, 1/2 tsp salt, garlic, rosemary, thyme, lemon zest and lemon juice.

• Pour this mixture over chicken. Place chicken in pan with vegetables. Bake in oven for 30 minutes.

• Stir chicken and vegetables and bake another 25 minutes, or until chicken is cooked through and vegetables are tender.

Shrimp and Black Bean Nachos

Ingredients

• 3/4 Cups cilantro,chopped

• 1/2 Cup red onion, diced

• 2 Tablespoons lemon juice

• 1 Tablespoon olive oil

• 1 Teaspoon Worcestershire Sauce

• 1/2 Teaspoon salt

• 1 Pound shrimp, peeled and cooked and chopped

• 2 Cups tomatoes, seeded, diced

* 1/2 Cup avocado, diced

* 15 Ounces black beans, drained and rinsed

* 1/2 Teaspoon cumin

* 4 Cups baked tortilla chips

Instructions

* Combine cilantro, onion, lime juice, oil, Worcestershire sauce, salt and shrimp in a large bowl; toss well.

* Cover and refrigerate for 30 minutes. Add tomato and avocado; stir well.

* Place the beans and cumin in a food processor, and process 30 seconds or until smooth.

* Spread each chip with 1-teaspoon black-bean mixture.

* Top with 1-tablespoon shrimp mixture. Serve

Southwestern Chicken Pitas

Ingredients

* 15 Ounces black beans, drained and rinsed

* 1/2 Cup red bell pepper, seeded and chopped

* 3 Tablespoons fresh lemon juice

- 2 Tablespoons fersh cilantro, minced

- 2 Teaspoons olive oil

- chicken breast halves, skinless

- round whole wheat pita pockets

- Monterrey Jack cheese, slices

Instructions

- In a bowl, combine beans, bell pepper, lime juice, and cilantro. Set aside.

- In a large pan, heat canola oil over medium-high heat. Cook chicken in pan until golden brown. Set aside for 10 without cutting.

- Warm pita bread in oven. Cut chicken into slices. For each sandwich, place cheese slice halves down center of one pita bread.

- Top with chicken breast slices and bean mixture. Roll up tightly. Cut in half and serve.

Spaghetti with Zucchini

Ingredients

- 1 Pound whole wheat spaghetti

- 2 zucchini, grated, water squeezed out or spiraled

- 2 Tablespoons butter

- 1 Tablespoon olive oil

- garlic cloves, minced

- 1/2 Cup Parmesan cheese, grated

Instructions

- Bring a large pot of salted water to boil. Add pasta and cook according to package directions until al dente.

- While pasta is cooking, in a large non-stick pan, heat butter and oil together. Add grated zucchini and cook for about 3 minutes. Add garlic and cook for one more minute, stirring constantly. Add 1/4 cup of grated parmesan cheese.

- Place pasta in a large shallow pasta bowl and toss in zucchini mixture. Top with remaining parmesan cheese. Serve

Spinach and Ham Pizza

Ingredients

- store bought baked thin crust whole wheat pizza shell

- 4 Cups baby spinach leaves, sliced thinly

- 1/2 Cup Mushrooms

- Tablespoons olive oil

- Ounces ham or prosciutto

- 1/4 Cup feta cheese, crumbled

- 1/4 Cup Parmesan cheese, grated

- Pieces garlic cloves, sliced thinly

Instructions

- Preheat oven to 450F degrees.

- Place the pizza shell on a cookie sheet. Scatter spinach and mushrooms all over crust. Drizzle with oil. Place ham or prosciutto, cheeses, and garlic on top of spinach & mushroom.

- Bake for 10-12 minutes, until crust is golden brown and spinach is wilted.

Summer Spaghetti

Ingredients

- 1 Pound whole wheat spaghetti

- 1/4 Cup olive oil

- shallot, minced

- garlic cloves, minced

- medium zucchini, chopped

• medium summer squash, chopped

• 1/4 Cup fresh basil, chopped

• 1/2 Teaspoon salt

• medium lemon, juiced

• 2 Tablespoons butter, room temperature

• freshly grated lemon peel

Instructions

• Bring a large pot of salted water to boil. Add pasta and cook according to package directions until al dente.

• In a large pan, heat oil over medium heat and cook the shallot and garlic stirring frequently.

• Add the zucchini, squash, and basil. Continue to cook, stirring occasionally, until all vegetables are tender. Season with salt and lemon juice.

• Immediately place the sautéed vegetables with all their juices in a large shallow pasta bowl.

• Add the linguine and butter, toss to mix well and serve immediately. Top with freshly grated lemon peel.

Tofu Stir Fry
Ingredients

- 14 Ounces firm tofu, drained, patted dry and cut into thick slices

- 1/4 Cup whole wheat flour

- 1 Tablespoon canola oil

- 1/2 Cup olive oil

- 2 Tablespoons balsamic vinegar

- 1 Tablespoon Dijon mustard

- 3 Tablespoons low sodium soy sauce

- 1/2 Cup onions, sliced

- 1/2 Cup carrots, sliced

- 1 Cup green beans, ends cut

- 1 Cup cabbage, chopped

- 1 Cup brown rice, cooked

Instructions

- In a shallow bowl or plate, mix tofu with flour until evenly coated. In a non-stick pan, heat canola oil over medium-high heat. Add tofu and cook until lightly brown. Remove from pan and put aside.

- Prepare dressing by whisking together olive oil, vinegar, mustard and soy sauce.

• In same pan, combine 2 tablespoons of the dressing mixture with onions, carrots, green beans, soy beans and cabbage.

• Stir fry for 10 minutes or until vegetables are tender. Add remaining dressing mixture and tofu. Mix. Cook for 2 minutes, stirring gently.

• Serve over hot brown rice.

Apple Chicken Pita Pocket

Ingredients

• 2 Cups chicken, cooked, cubed

• 2 apples, unpeeled, chopped

• celery stalk, chopped

• 1/3 Cup plain yogurt

• 1/4 Cup mayonaise

• 4 round whole wheat pita breads

• 4 romaine lettuce leaves

Instructions

• In a medium bowl, combine the chicken, apples, and celery.

- Add yogurt and mayonnaise. Mix well. Slice pita to make a pocket.

- Line with lettuce leaf and fill pita pocket with 1 cup of mixture per pita bread.

- Serve with mixed fruit salad (no berries).

Aromatic Rice with Lentils

Ingredients

- 2 Tablespoons olive oil

- onion, chopped

- carrots, chopped

- red bell pepper, seeded and chopped

- garlic cloves, minced

- 1 Tablespoon fresh basil, chopped

- 1 Tablespoon fresh oregano, chopped

- 1/2 Tablespoon fresh sage, chopped

- 1 Cup brown rice

- Cups chicken broth

- 1 Cup lentils, uncooked and rinsed

Instructions

• In a large pan, heat olive oil over medium-high heat. Cook onion, carrot and pepper until softened, about 5-7 minutes.

• Add garlic and cook for one more minute. Add basil, oregano, sage and rice. Stir to combine.

• Stir in broth. Bring to a boil, stirring occasionally. Add lentils. Cover and reduce heat to low and let simmer for 20-25 minutes.

• Fluff with fork and serve.

Bean and Mushroom Stew

Ingredients

• 2 Tablespoons olive oil

• 1 Pound white mushrooms, sliced

• 1 Cup onion, chopped

• 1 Teaspoon garlic cloves, minced

• 3/4 Teaspoons dried thyme

• 28 Ounces chicken broth

• 14 Ounces can stewed tomatoes, chopped

• 1/4 Cup white wine, optional

• 30 Ounces can,cannellini beans, drained and rinsed

Instructions

• In a large saucepan, heat olive oil over medium high heat. Cook mushrooms, onion, garlic and thyme until onion is tender and mushrooms are slightly golden (about 7 minutes).

• Add chicken broth, tomatoes and wine and bring to a boil. Cover and simmer for about 35 additional minutes.

• In a small bowl, mash 1 cup of the beans until smooth; add to stew. Stir in remaining beans, heat until hot.

• Serve immediately with a side of cooked long grain rice, if desired.

Bean and Vegetable Casserole

Ingredients

• 3 Tablespoons vegetable oil

• large onion, chopped

• celery stalks, chopped

• medium green pepper, seeded and diced

• medium tomatoes, seeded and chopped

• Cups red kidney beans, drained and rinsed

• 1 Cup cannellini beans, drained and rinsed

- 1 Cup barley

- 2/3 Cups Italian parsley, chopped

- 1/2 Teaspoon salt

- 1 Teaspoon Italian seasoning

- 1 Teaspoon cumin

- 1 3/4 Cup boiling water

Instructions

- Preheat oven to 350F degrees.

- In a large non-stick pan, heat oil over medium-high heat. Add onion, celery, and green pepper. Cook for 10 minutes or until vegetables soften.

- Stir in tomatoes, kidney beans, cannellini beans, barley, parsley, salt, Italian seasoning, and cumin.

- Transfer mixture to a 2-to 3 quart casserole that has been sprayed with non-stick cooking spray.

- Add boiling water. Cover. Bake at 350 degrees for 1-1/2 hours or until barley is tender and liquid is absorbed.

Bean Enchiladas

Ingredients

- 14 Ounces can red beans, drained, rinsed, mashed

- 2 Cups cheddar cheese, grated

- 1/2 Cup onion, chopped

- 1/4 Cup black olives, sliced

- 2 Cups tomato sauce

- 2 Teaspoons garlic salt

- 8 whole wheat tortillas

Instructions

- Preheat oven to 350F degrees.

- In a medium bowl, combine the mashed beans, cheese, onions, olives, one cup tomato sauce, and garlic salt.

- Place about 1/3 cup bean mixture along center of each tortilla. Roll up and place enchiladas in large baking dish.

- Spoon remaining tomato sauce on top of the filled tortillas. Sprinkle with additional cheese, if desired.

- Bake for 15 to 20 minutes or until thoroughly heated.

Beef and Penne Pasta Toss
Ingredients

- 1 Pound whole wheat penne pasta

- 1 Pound ground beef, lean

- 2 Tablespoons olive oil

- small onion, chopped

- garlic cloves, minced

- 15 Ounces can tomatoes, seeded, diced

- Cups medium zucchini, seeded, chopped

- 8 Ounces fresh spinach, chopped

- 1 Cup Parmesan cheese, grated

Instructions

- Bring a large pot of salted water to a boil. Cook penne pasta al dente according to package directions.

- In a large non-stick pan, brown ground beef over medium-high heat for 6 to 8 minutes, breaking up any large pieces. Remove beef and set aside on paper towels to drain excess fat.

- In the same pan, heat olive oil over medium-high heat. Cook onions and garlic for about 5 minutes or until soft. Add tomatoes and zucchini and continue cooking 5 minutes more. Add spinach and cook until it just wilts, 2-3 minutes.

• Return beef to skillet and stir in 1/2 cup cheese; heat through Transfer pasta to a large serving bowl and spoon meat mixture on top.

• Toss until well combined and sprinkle with remaining cheese.

Beef Fajitas

Ingredients

• 6 Ounces flank steak, trimmed of fat

• 2 Teaspoons lime juice

• 1 Teaspoon garlic, chopped

• 1 Teaspoon olive oil, divided

• 15 Ounces can red beans, drained, rinsed, mashed

• 1/2 Cup medium green pepper, seeded and thinly sliced

• 1/2 Cup red bell pepper, thinly sliced

• 1 Tablespoon scallions, chopped

• 4 whole wheat tortillas

Instructions

• Season flank steak with salt. Let sit for 10 minutes. Grill flank steak over high heat until cooked on both sides. Place steak on separate plate to rest for 10 minutes. Cut flank steak into thin strips against the grain.

• In a small bowl, whisk together lime juice, garlic, and 1/2 teaspoon of olive oil. Set aside.

• In a small pan, heat the other 1/2 tsp olive oil and combine beans, bell peppers and scallions and heat through.

• To assemble fajitas, take tortilla and place steak inside. Top with bean mixture and drizzle some of the lime sauce on top.

• Roll into fajita and serve immediately.

Black Bean Quesadillas

Ingredients

• 1 Tablespoon olive oil

• 1/2 small onion, chopped

• 1/2 Cup red bell pepper, seeded, chopped

• clove, minced

• 28 Ounces black beans, rinsed, drained, lightly mashed

• 1/2 Teaspoon cumin

• Tablespoons cilantro, chopped

• 1/4 Cup black olives, sliced

• Cups fresh spinach, chopped

* 3/4 Cups Monterey Jack cheese, shredded

* 8 whole wheat tortillas

Instructions

* Preheat oven to 350 degrees.

* In a medium pan, heat olive oil over medium heat. Cook onions and red peppers until soft, about 5 minutes. Add garlic and continue to cook another 2 minutes, add mashed beans, cilantro and olives, and cumin and cook another 5 minutes to combine all ingredients.

* Spread mixture evenly onto 4 tortillas. Sprinkle with spinach and cheese.

* Top with remaining tortillas. Bake tortillas on ungreased cookie sheet for 12 minutes. Cut into wedges and serve.

Broccoli and Mushroom Brown Rice

Ingredients

* 1 Tablespoon olive oil

* medium onion, chopped

* garlic cloves, minced

* 1 Cup instant brown rice

* 8 Ounces Portobello mushrooms, sliced

• 3/4 Cups vegetable broth

• 1 Pound broccoli florets, fresh, cut into bite-size pieces

• 1/2 Teaspoon salt

• 1/4 Teaspoon pepper

Instructions

• In a medium pan, heat olive oil over medium-high heat. Cook onions and garlic until translucent, about 5 minutes.

• Stir in rice and mushrooms and cook 3-5 minutes or until mushrooms have released all of their juices. Add the broth and bring to a boil. Reduce heat to medium-low and cover until liquid is absorbed (about 7 - 8 minutes).

• Place broccoli florets in a microwave-safe casserole dish and sprinkle with salt and pepper and add 4 tbs. water. Cover and cook at high power for 5 to 7 minutes or until tender.

• Fluff rice with a fork and pour into a serving platter and top with broccoli. Toss to combine and serve. Can be topped with freshly grated Parmesan cheese and fresh Italian parsley.

Chicken and Asparagus Pasta

Ingredients

• 1 Pound whole wheat penne pasta

• 2 Tablespoons olive oil

• 1 Pound   chicken breast halves, boneless and sliced into strips

• 1/2 Teaspoon poultry seasoning

• 4 Pieces garlic cloves, minced

• 1 1/2 Cup asparagus, frozen, thawed, cut into 1 inch pieces

• 1 Cup peas, frozen, thawed

• 1/4 Cup Parmesan cheese, grated

Instructions

• Bring a large pot of salted water to boil. Add pasta and cook al dente according to package directions.

• Heat one tablespoon olive oil in a pan over medium heat and cook chicken with poultry seasoning until golden. Remove cooked chicken from the pan.

• Add the remaining tablespoon of olive oil, garlic, asparagus and peas. Cook until vegetables are tender.

• Place chicken back in with the asparagus mixture and cook together for 2 minutes or until heated through.

• Place pasta in a large shallow pasta bowl and toss with chicken mixture. Top with parmesan cheese.

Chicken and Avocado Pitas

Ingredients

* 2 Cups cooked chicken. chopped

* avocado, medium, chopped

* 14 Ounces can red beans, drained, rinsed, mashed

* 1 Teaspoon lemon juice

* 1 Cup tomatoes, seeded, chopped

* 1 Cup cottage cheese

* 4 whole wheat pita pockets

Instructions

* In a large mixing bowl, combine chicken, avocado, red beans, lemon juice, tomatoes, and cottage cheese.

* Slice the pita bread to make a pocket and spoon in the chicken mixture. Serve.

Chicken and Lentil Pita

Ingredients

* 1 Cup cream cheese

* 1 Tablespoon mayonnaise

- 2 Cups cooked chicken. chopped

- 1 Cup tomatoes, seeded, diced

- 14 Ounces can lentils, cooked

- 4 Cups Romaine lettuce leaves

- 2 Cups alfalfa sprouts

- 4 whole wheat pita pockets

Instructions

- In a medium bowl, combine cream cheese and mayonnaise until well blended.

- Add chicken, tomatoes, lentils; mix well.

- Cut the top of each pita bread. Place lettuce inside and fill each pita with the chicken mixture.

- Top with alfalfa sprouts. Serve.

Chicken Florentine

Ingredients

- 2 Tablespoons olive oil

- 2 zucchinis, seeded, thinly sliced

- 1/2 Cup green onion, sliced

- 2 chicken breast, cubed

- 1/2 Teaspoon salt

- 1/2 Teaspoon thyme, ground

- 3 Cups long grain rice, cooked

- 4 Cups fresh spinach, chopped

- 1/4 Cup Parmesan cheese, grated

Instructions

- In a medium pan, heat olive oil over medium heat.

- Add zucchini, onions, and chicken, stirring occasionally for 5 to 10 minutes, or until chicken is golden.

- Add salt, thyme, rice and spinach. Cook and stir for another 6 - 8 minutes or until heated through and spinach wilts.

- Remove from heat, transfer to a large serving bowl, and stir in cheese. Serve.

Chipotle Black Bean Chili

Ingredients

- 1 Tablespoon olive oil

- 1 Cup onion, finely chopped

- garlic cloves, minced

- 1/2 Teaspoon chipotle powder

- 1/2 Teaspoon cumin

- 1/4 Teaspoon salt

- 30 Ounces can black beans, drained and rinsed

- 28 Ounces tomatoes, seeded, chopped

- 1 Teaspoon fresh cilantro

Instructions

- In a large non-stick pan, heat olive oil over medium heat.

- Add onions and garlic and cook 5 minutes or until they are soft. Add chipotle powder, cumin, salt, beans, and tomatoes bring to a boil.

- Reduce heat, cover and simmer 15-25 or until chili thickens.

- Garnish with fresh cilantro.

Cottage Crunch Wraps

Ingredients

- 3/4 Cups cottage cheese

- 1/4 Cup carrots, shredded

- green onion, sliced

- 1/2 Cup tomatoes, seeded, chopped

- 1/2 Cup cabbage, chopped

- 1 Teaspoon lime juice

- whole wheat tortillas

Instructions

- In a medium bowl, place cheese, carrots, onions, tomatoes, and cabbage and mix well. Add lime juice. Place mixture in tortillas, wrap and serve.

Couscous with Chicken

Ingredients

- 4 Tablespoons olive oil

- 1 Pound chicken thighs, sliced into strips

- onion, chopped

- garlic cloves, minced

- 1 Cup carrots, shredded

- 1 Teaspoon smoked paprika

- 1 Teaspoon cumin

- 1/8 Teaspoon cinnamon

- 1/2 Teaspoon salt

- 1 Cup dried fruits, chopped (apricots, dates)

- 4 Cups chicken broth

- 2 Tablespoons butter

- 1 1/2 Cup couscous

- 1/2 Cup Italian parsley, chopped

Instructions

- In a large, deep pan, heat oil over medium-high heat.

- Cook chicken and brown 3 to 4 minutes on each side. Add onions, garlic, carrots, and season with spices and salt. Cook 6-8 minutes.

- Stir the fruits into the chicken and vegetables, and 2 1/2 cups of stock. Allow to boil. Reduce heat to low, cover and simmer 10 minutes.

- In a separate small saucepan, over medium heat, pour 1 1/2 cups stock and bring up to a boil then stir in couscous.

- Remove from heat, cover and let stand 5 minutes. Fluff with fork and serve with chicken.

Couscous with Vegetables

Ingredients

- 1 1/2 Cup chicken broth

- 1 Cup couscous

- 4 Tablespoons olive oil, divided

- red onion, chopped

- garlic cloves, minced

- tomatoes, seeded, chopped

- yellow bell pepper, seeded and chopped

- red bell pepper, seeded and chopped

- zucchinis, seeded, chopped

- 1 Cup peas, thawed from frozen

- 2 Tablespoons balsamic vinegar

- 2 Tablespoons Feta cheese, crumbled

Instructions

- In a medium saucepan, over high heat, bring chicken broth and 1 tbs of olive oil to a boil. Remove from heat and stir in couscous. Cover and let sit for 5-10 minutes.

• In a separate pan over medium heat, add the remaining oil and cook the onions and garlic until softened.

• Mix in the tomatoes, bell peppers and zucchinis. Cook and stir until tender.

• Add peas and cook 2-3 more minutes. Add vinegar and cheese and toss to combine.

• Spoon vegetable mixture over couscous. Serve.

Easy Beef Stir Fry

Ingredients

• 1/4 Cup orange juice

• 1/4 Cup low-sodium soy sauce

• 2 Tablespoons rice vinegar

• 1/4 Cup water

• 2 Tablespoons canola oil

• 8 Ounces beef round tip steak, thinly sliced

• garlic cloves, minced

• 6 Ounces peas, thawed from frozen

• bunch broccoli florets

• 8 Ounces edamame, shelled

• 1 1/2 Teaspoon cornstarch, dissolved in 1/4 C warm water

Instructions

• In a small bowl, combine orange juice, soy sauce, rice vinegar, and water until well combined. Set aside.

• In a large non-stick pan, heat 1 tablespoon of canola oil over medium-high heat. Add the beef and cook, stirring, until just browned, about 2 minutes. Transfer the beef to a separate plate.

• Heat another tablespoon of oil over medium heat and cook garlic about 1 minute, without burning it. Add peas, broccoli and edamame, and continue to cook for 3 minutes.

• Add the soy sauce mixture and cook, stirring, until broccoli is cooked and crisp-tender, about 5 minutes.

• Add the sliced beef back into pan and add dissolved cornstarch in water and stir to combine all ingredients.

• Cook until mixture thickens slightly and beef is heated through. Serve immediately.

Easy Turkey Chili

Ingredients

• 3 Tablespoons olive oil

• garlic cloves, minced

- onion, chopped

- 1 Pound ground turkey

- Bay leaf

- 1 Teaspoon ground cumin

- 1 Teaspoon dried oregano

- tomato, seeded, chopped

- 14 Ounces can tomato sauce

- 1 Cup beef broth

- 1 Teaspoon salt

- 28 Ounces can red beans, drained and rinsed

Instructions

- In a large pot, heat oil over medium heat and cook garlic and onions for a 5 minutes.

- Increase heat to high and add turkey, bay leaf, cumin and oregano. Cook until turkey has browned, about 5-7 minutes.

- Add tomato, tomato sauce, broth and salt. Bring pot to a boil and then lower heat to simmer. Cover and simmer for about 20 minutes.

- Add beans and more water if needed, and continue to simmer for 25 more minutes. Serve.

Garbanzo Pita Pockets

Ingredients

• 15 Ounces can garbanzo beans, drained, rinsed

• 6 Ounces   can artichokes, marinated, quartered, liquid reserved

• 1 Tablespoon black olives. sliced

• 1 Tablespoon green olives, sliced

• green bell pepper, seeded, chopped

• red bell pepper, seeded and chopped

• small red onion, thinly sliced

• 2 Tablespoons red wine vinegar

• 1/2 Cup fresh basil, chopped

• whole wheat pita pockets

Instructions

• In a large bowl, combine the garbanzo beans, artichokes and their liquid, olives, garlic, peppers, onion, vinegar and basil. Mix well and set aside.

• Slice pita bread to make a pocket. Place a lettuce leaf in each pita and fill with the garbanzo filling. Serve.

74

Ingredients

- 1/4 Teaspoon salt

- lemon, juiced

- 2 Tablespoons olive oil

- fish filets, trout or tilapia

- 1/2 Cup red onion, chopped

- 1/2 Cup jicama, peeled, chopped

- 1/3 Cup red bell pepper, seeded and chopped

- 2/3 Cups fresh cilantro, finely chopped

- 1 Cup black beans, drained, rinsed

- lime, zest and juice

- 1 Tablespoon plain yogurt

- whole wheat tortillas

Instructions

- In a small bowl, combine salt, lemon juice, and olive oil. Pour mixture over fish fillets and let marinate for 10 minutes.

• Grill fish over high heat until cooked through, about 3 minutes per side.

• In a separate bowl, combine onion, jicama, bell pepper, cilantro, beans, zest and juice of lime and yogurt to make a "salsa".

• To make tacos, place fish in warmed tortilla and cover with "salsa" and fold in half. Serve.

Grilled Steak with Spinach and Apple Salad

Ingredients

• beef steaks, rib-eye or sirloin

• 4 Tablespoons olive oil

• salt and pepper to taste

• 1 Tablespoon balsamic vinegar

• 2 Cups fresh baby spinach, washed and dried

• apple (preferably tart, like Granny Smith), unpeeled and sliced

• 4 Ounces Parmesan cheese, grated

Instructions

• Prepare steaks for grill by pouring 2 tbs olive oil and salt to taste. Grill over high heat to desired doneness, about 7 minutes per side for medium. Once cooked, place steaks on plate to rest and let juices redistribute without cutting.

• To make dressing, in a small bowl, whisk together balsamic vinegar, 2 tbs olive oil and salt and pepper to taste.

• On individual plates, stack spinach, apples and steak that have been cut diagonally. Drizzle with dressing and top with Parmesan cheese.

Grilled Vegetable Quesadilla

Ingredients

• zucchini, sliced in half, lengthwise

• yello squash, sliced in half lengthwise

• onion, sliced in fourths, lenghtwise

• red pepper, seeded and quartered

• Portobello mushroom cap

• 1/2 Teaspoon Italian seasoning

• 1/4 Teaspoon salt

• whole wheat tortillas

• 1/2 Cup Mozzarella cheese, shredded

Instructions

• Grill vegetables over medium heat until all of the vegetables are cooked. Season with Italian seasoning and salt. Slice vegetables and toss together.

• Heat a pan sprayed with non-stick cooking spray over medium heat and place one tortilla in the pan. Spread some of the vegetable mixture over the tortilla, sprinkle with cheese and top with the remaining tortilla. Turn tortilla over and heat the other side until cheese melts but do not brown the tortillas. Serve.

Grilled Veggie Sandwich

Ingredients

• eggplant, sliced in half-inch thick slices

• zucchini, sliced in half-inch thick slices

• red pepper, seeded and quartered

• portobello mushroom caps

• 1/2 Cup olive oil

• 1/4 Teaspoon salt

• 1 Cup goat cheese

• 8 Ounces whole wheat crusty bread like baguette

• 1 Cup fresh baby spinach, washed and dried

Instructions

• With a pastry brush, brush olive oil on the vegetable slices and the mushrooms caps. Season them with salt.

• Place vegetables on a hot grill and cook until they are tender. To assemble, slice mushrooms into 1/4-inch slices, spread both sides of the bread with goat cheese and then top with 1 slice each of grilled vegetables and a quarter of the mushrooms.

• Top with spinach and remaining piece of bread. Serve.

Lentil Linguine Stew

Ingredients

• 3 Tablespoons olive oil

• onion, chopped

• garlic cloves, minced

• carrots, chopped

• celery stalks, chopped

• 1 Cup lentils, uncooked, rinsed

• 6 Cups vegetable broth

• 4 Cups water

• 2 Teaspoons salt

• bay leaves

• 1/2 Cup linguine, cut into 1-inch pieces

• 2 Cups kale, chopped

• 1/2 Cup Italian parsley, chopped

Instructions

• In a large pot, heat olive oil over moderate heat. Cook the onion, garlic, and carrots and celery for 10 minutes, stirring occasionally, until tender.

• Add the lentils, broth, water, salt, and bay leaf to the pot. Bring to a boil. Reduce the heat and simmer, partially covered, stirring occasionally, for 25 minutes.

• Add the linguine and simmer, stirring occasionally, until the lentils are tender and the pasta and kale are tender, 15 to 20 minutes longer.

• Stir parsley into the stew. Serve.

Lentil Risotto

Ingredients

• 2 Tablespoons olive oil

• medium leeks, chopped

• garlic cloves, minced

• red bell pepper, seeded and chopped

• 3 Cups chicken broth

• 1 1/4 Cup long grain rice

• 1 Tablespoon fresh basil, chopped

• 1 Cup lentils, cooked

• 1/4 Cup Italian parsley, chopped

• 1/4 Cup Parmesan cheese, grated

Instructions

• In a large pot, heat olive oil over moderate heat and cook leeks, garlic, and red pepper until softened.

• Add broth along with the rice, and basil. Cover and let simmer until rice is done then add cooked lentils and stir for 10 minutes.

• Remove from heat and add parsley and parmesan cheese. Serve.

Lentil Stew
ingredients

• 1 Tablespoon vegetable oil

• onion, chopped

81

- garlic cloves, minced

- green bell pepper, seeded, chopped

- Cups kale, chopped

- Cups vegetable broth

- 1 1/4 Cup lentils, uncooked, rinsed

- 15 Ounces can tomato sauce

- 1 Tablespoon Italian seasoning

- 1/2 Teaspoon paprika

Instructions

- In a large saucepan, heat oil over medium-high heat. Cook onion, garlic, and bell pepper, stirring frequently, until vegetables are tender.

- Stir in water, lentils, tomato sauce and spices. Reduce heat to low and partially cover and simmer 35 to 40 minutes or until lentils are tender. Serve.

Ziti with Zesty Chicken

Ingredients

- 1 Pound whole wheat ziti pasta or bowtie pasta

- 2 Teaspoons olive oil

- onion, chopped

- 1 Tablespoon Dijon mustard

- Tablespoons whole wheat flour

- Cups chicken broth

- 1/4 Cup lemon juice

- 12 Ounces frozen peas, thawed

- 1/4 Cup fresh Italian parsley, chopped

- 12 Ounces cooked chicken, chopped

Instructions

- Bring a large pot of salted water to a boil. Add pasta and cook according to package instructions until al dente. Drain.

- While pasta is cooking, in a large non-stick pan, heat olive oil over medium heat. Add the onion and cook for 3 minutes. Stir in the Dijon mustard and flour. Gradually whisk in the chicken broth, stirring constantly to avoid clumps.

- Bring the broth to a boil and stir in the lemon juice, peas and parsley. Add cooked pasta and cooked chicken to sauce and serve.

Vegeterian Penne Pasta

Ingredients

- 1/2 Pound whole wheat penne or bowtie pasta

- 1 Tablespoon salt

- 2 Tablespoons olive oil

- 8 Ounces white mushrooms, sliced

- 8 Ounces asparagus, chopped

- 8 Ounces red bell pepper, seeded and chopped

- 1/4 Cup Parmesan cheese, grated

- 1/4 Cup fresh basil, chopped

Instructions

- Bring a large pot of salted water to boil. Add pasta and cook according to package directions until al dente. Drain.

- While the pasta is cooking, in a medium non-stick pan, heat olive oil over medium heat. Add the mushrooms and cook for about five minutes to release all the water.

- Add the asparagus and bell pepper and sauté for 3-4 minutes, until softened. Add cooked pasta to pan and add Parmesan cheese, stir until well combined.

- Transfer to a serving bowl, garnish with fresh basil and serve.

Ingredients

- 1 Cup sugar snap peas

- 2 Tablespoons olive oil

- onion, chopped

- 8 Ounces mushrooms, sliced

- 8 Ounces artichoke hearts, drained, chopped

- 8 Ounces green lentils, drained

- 4 Tablespoons half and half

- 1/2 Teaspoon salt

- 1/2 Teaspoon pepper

Instructions

- Bring a small sauce pan of salted water to boil. Add sugar snap peas and turn off heat and set aside for 4 minutes until tender. Drain under cold water and pat dry with paper towel. Set aside.

- In a medium pan, heat olive oil and cook onions for 3-5 minutes. Add sliced mushrooms and stir for 2-3 minutes. Add the sugar snap peas, artichoke hearts, and lentils to the pan. Stir-fry for 2 minutes.

- Stir in the cream and salt and pepper and cook for 1 minute. Serve.

Ingredients

- 2 Tablespoons vegetable oil

- onion, sliced

- Tablespoons curry powder

- 1/2 Teaspoon garlic powder

- 1/4 Teaspoon fresh ginger, grated

- 15 Ounces tomatoes, seeded and chopped

- 30 Ounces garbanzo beans, not drained

- Cups potatoes, unpeeled, chopped

- 1 Cup carrots, sliced

- 2 Cups cauliflower, chopped

- 10 Ounces frozen peas, thawed

- 1/4 Teaspoon salt

- 1/4 Teaspoon pepper

Instructions

• In a large non-stick pan, heat oil over medium-high heat. Cook onions until softened. Add curry powder, garlic powder and ginger; cook 2 minutes.

• Add tomatoes, garbanzo beans, potatoes, and carrots and stir together. Add cauliflower, cover and reduce heat to simmer. Cook for 20-30 minutes, until vegetable are tender, adding water if necessary. Stir in peas and salt and pepper; cook 5 more minutes.

• Serve over hot rice.

Vegetable and Butternut Squash Curry

Ingredients

• 1 1/2 Pound butternut squash, seeded, peeled and chopped

• 1 Tablespoon olive oil

• onion, finely chopped

• 1 Tablespoon curry powder

• 1 2/3 Cup coconut milk

• 1 Cup water

• 3 Cups fresh spinach, chopped

• 14 Ounces butter beans, drained and rinsed

• 2 Tablespoons cilantro, chopped

Instructions

• In a small saucepan, place squash and cover with water. Boil squash until tender and drain.

• In a large pan, heat olive oil and cook onions until tender. Stir in curry powder, continue stirring until fragrant, about 3 minutes. Stir in coconut milk and water. Bring to boil; simmer, uncovered, about five minutes or until the mixture just thickens.

• Add squash, spinach, butter beans and cilantro. Stir until heated through. Serve.

Turkey and Barley Casserole

Ingredients

• 1 Pound ground turkey

• 1/2 Teaspoon salt

• small onion, chopped

• carrots, chopped

• celery stalks, chopped

• green bell pepper, seeded and chopped

• white button mushrooms, quartered

• 2 1/2 Cups chicken broth

* 1 Cup barley

* 1 Tablespoon poultry seasoning

* bay leaf

Instructions

* Preheat oven to 375F degrees.

* In a large pan, over medium- high heat, cook ground turkey with salt until browned, about 5 minutes.

* Add onions, carrots, celery and green peppers. Cook until tender, about 5 minutes. Add mushrooms, stock, barley, poultry seasoning and bay leaf.

* Mix together and place mixture in a 9x13 inch baking dish. Cover and bake in the preheated oven for 1 hour. Serve.

Tuna Cakes and Smashed Potatoes

Ingredients

* potatoes, unpeeled, chopped

* 2 Teaspoons salt

* 1/2 Cup milk

* 3 Tablespoons butter

* 3 Tablespoons canola oil

89

- 12 Ounces tuna fish, drained

- egg, beaten

- 2 Tablespoons green onions, diced

- 1/4 Cup mayonnaise

- 1/2 Cup whole wheat bread, cut into small pieces

- lemon juice, optional

Instructions

- Cook potatoes in a small saucepan until tender. Drain. Place potatoes back in pan. Heat the milk and butter in microwave until hot. With a potato masher, roughly smash the potatoes while adding hot liquid until combined and set aside.

- In a bowl, combine tuna, egg, green onions, mayonnaise, bread crumbs, and lemon juice. Form into patties. Allow to refrigerate and become firm for 10 minutes.

- Heat oil over medium-high heat, cook patties until golden brown, about 2 minutes on each side. Serve with potatoes.

Tortellini with Navy Bean Sauce
Ingredients

- 2 Cups navy or white beans, dry, uncooked

- 2 Tablespoons olive oil

- small onion, chopped

- garlic cloves, minced

- 1 Cup tomatoes, seeded and chopped

- 2 Tablespoons tomato paste

- 7 Cups chicken broth

- bay leaf

- 1 Pound tortellini, store bought, filling of your choice

- 1/4 Cup fresh basil, chopped

Instructions

- Cover the beans with water and soak for at least 8 hours or overnight. Drain.

- In a non-stick pan, heat olive oil over medium heat. Add the onion and cook, for 3 minutes. Mix in the garlic and cook for another minute. Add the tomatoes and tomato paste, stir and cook for a few minutes. Add chicken broth, bay leaf and beans and bring to a boil, reduce the heat and simmer, uncovered, for 1 1/2 hours.

- Pour the bean mixture into a blender or food processor and process into a puree. Adjust the consistency with more stock if necessary.

• Bring large pot of salted water to boil. Cook tortellini according to package directions.

• Pour sauce over tortellini garnish with basil and serve.

Beans with Greens Soup

Ingredients

• 2 Tablespoons olive oil

• onion, chopped

• 4 garlic cloves, minced

• celery stalks, sliced finely

• carrots, sliced

• 6 Cups chicken broth

• 1/4 Teaspoon thyme

• 1/4 Teaspoon rosemary

• bay leaf

• 14 Ounces cannellini beans, drained and rinsed

• 1/2 Teaspoon salt

• 1 Cup leafy greens (kale, spinach or chard), chopped

Instructions

• In a large soup pot, heat olive oil over medium heat. Add onions and cook until softened, about 3 minutes. Stir in onion, garlic, celery, and carrots and continue to cook for 5 minutes, stirring occasionally.

• Add chicken broth, thyme, rosemary, and bay leaf and cook until it comes to a boil. Reduce heat and cover and simmer gently for about 45-60 minutes.

• Add beans and season with salt. Add leafy greens and cook until tender, approximately 5-10 minutes, depending on the greens being used. Serve.

• For a creamier texture, prior to adding the greens, the broth and vegetables can be blended with an immersion blender until desired consistency is reached.

Beef and Vegetable Soup

Ingredients

• 1/2 Pound stew beef, diced

• 1/2 bag frozen vegetable medley

• 1/4 Cup barley

• 32 Ounces beef broth

• 2 tomatoes, seeded and chopped

• 1 Teaspoon garlic powder

- 1 Teaspoon paprika

- 1 Teaspoon oregano

- bay leaf

- yellow or red potato, chopped

Instructions

- In a large soup pot, over medium-high heat, brown ground beef.

- Add frozen vegetables, barley, broth, tomatoes, garlic powder, paprika, oregano and bay leaf. Bring the pot to a boil, Reduce heat, cover and simmer for 15 minutes.

- Add the potatoes and allow to simmer again for another 20 minutes or until they are tender.

Cannellini and Butter Bean Soup
Ingredients

- 1 Tablespoon olive oil

- 3 slices pancetta, chopped

- 3 garlic cloves, minced

- 2 medium onions, chopped

- 28 Ounces cannellini beans, drained and rinsed

- 28 Ounces butter (lima) beans, drained and rinsed

- 2 Teaspoons thyme, fresh, chopped

- 1 Tablespoon balsamic vinegar

- 6 Cups vegetable stock

Instructions

- In a large soup pot, heat olive oil over medium-high heat. Cook pancetta until crisp.

- Add garlic and onions. Cook until onions are tender, about 5 minutes.

- Stir in beans, thyme, vinegar and vegetable stock. Bring pot to a boil, reduce heat and simmer uncovered for 25 minutes. Serve.

Chicken and Split Pea Soup

Ingredients

- 1 Pound skinless, boneless, chicken breast, cubed

- 2 Tablespoons olive oil

- 2 lage onions, chopped

- 3 garlic cloves, minced

- 3 carrots, chopped

* bay leaf

* 1 Teaspoon salt

* 1 Teaspoon poultry seasoning

* 8 Cups chicken broth

* 1/2 Cup dried split peas, washed and drained

* 1 Cup peas, thawed if frozen

Instructions

* In a large soup pot, heat olive oil over medium heat.

* Add chicken and cook for 5 minutes, until lightly browned. Add onions, garlic, carrots, bay leaf, salt and seasoning and cook until vegetables soften, stirring occasionally.

* Add broth and split peas to pot and bring to a boil. Reduce heat, cover and simmer on low heat for 30-45 minutes.

* To the soup, add green peas and heat for 5 minutes, stirring to combine all ingredients.

Creamy Carrot Soup

Ingredients

* 2 Tablespoons olive oil

* 4 Cups carrots, chopped

* onion, chopped

* garlic cloves, minced

* 1 Tablespoon curry powder

* Cups chicken broth

* 1 1/2 Cup carrot juice

Instructions

* In a large soup pot, heat oil over medium heat.

* Add carrots and onion and continue to cook for about 6-8 minutes. Add garlic and curry powder and cook for another minute.

* Next, add broth and 1/2 tsp salt and simmer over low heat. Cover and let simmer for about 15 minutes.

* Add carrot juice and mix well. Puree the soup in a blender, working in batches. Return the soup to the pan and season with salt and pepper. Serve.

* Note: for a richer texture, some cream can be mixed in.

Creamy Chickpea Soup

Ingredients

* 2 1/2 Cups vegetable broth

- 2 Cups fresh baby spinach

- 2 Cups tomatoes, seeded and chopped

- 2 Cups hummus, homemade or store bought

- 1 Tablespoon lemon juice

Instructions

- In a medium pot, bring vegetable broth to a boil.

- Add spinach and tomatoes and cook until spinach wilts, about 4 – 5 minutes.

- Lower heat and stir in the hummus and lemon juice and cook until heated through.

Split Pea Soup

Ingredients

- 1 Tablespoon olive oil

- onion, chopped

- celery stalk, chopped

- carrot, chopped

- red bell pepper, seeded, chopped

- 1 Cup yellow split peas, uncooked, rinsed

- 1/2 Cups chicken broth

- Cups water

- 1/4 Cup plain yogurt

Instructions

- In a large soup pot, heat olive oil over medium-high heat.

- Add onion, celery, carrot, and red peppers. Cook for 7 -8 minutes or until tender.

- Add split peas, chicken broth and water, bring to a boil. Reduce heat to low and let simmer, covered for 45 minutes or until peas have fallen apart.

- Puree soup a hand blender until smooth. Garnish with a dollop of yogurt if desired. Serve.

Smooth Broccoli Soup

Ingredients

- 2 Tablespoons olive oil

- leek, choppped

- celery stalk, chopped

- garlic cloves, minced

- small potatoes, unpeeled, chopped

- 1/2 Teaspoon salt

- bay leaf

- Cups vegetable broth

- 1 1/2 Cup broccoli florets

Instructions

- In a large soup pan, heat oil over medium-high heat. Cook leek, celery, garlic, potatoes, salt and bay leaf until lightly browned.

- Add stock and bring to a boil. Reduce heat, cover and simmer 30 minutes.

- Add broccoli florets to pot and bring back to a boil. Reduce heat, cover, and simmer another 15 minutes or until all vegetables are tender.

- Remove from heat and let cool. Remove bay leaf. Puree soup with a hand blender, until smooth. Serve.

Slow Cooker Lentil, Sausage and Kale Soup
Ingredients

- 2 Tablespoons olive oil

- 1 Pound Italian seasoned turkey sausage, casings removed

- onion, chopped

• carrots, chopped

• celery stalks, chopped

• 1 Teaspoon Italian seasoning

• 1/2 Teaspoon black pepper

• 2 garlic cloves, chopped

• 15 Ounces diced tomatoes

• 1 1/2 Cup green or brown lentils

• Cups vegetable or chicken broth

• 3 Cups kale, chopped roughly

Instructions

• In a slow cooker, heat the olive oil and brown/sear the Italian turkey sausage, crumbling with a wooden spoon.

• Add onions, carrots, celery, and Italian seasoning and pepper, and cook until vegetables soften about 5-7 minutes. Add garlic and cook another minute.

• Add tomatoes, lentils, and broth and stir to combine all ingredients.

• Cook covered on low for 6-8 hours, until lentils get tender, not mushy.

• Add kale and stir and cook until kale wilts. Adjust seasoning.

• Serve with grated Parmesan on top if desired and crusty whole-wheat bread.

• Note- If the slow cooker does not have a sear/browning function, the sausage and vegetables and seasonings can be cooked in a separate skillet and then added to the slow cooker.

Kidney Bean Salsa

Ingredients

• 14 Ounces red kidney beans, drained and rinsed

• 2 tomatoes, seeded and chopped

• yellow bell pepper, seeded and chopped

• avocado, chopped

• 1 Tablespoon cilantro, chopped

• Tablespoons lime juice

• 1/4 Teaspoon salt

Instructions

- In large bowl, mix all ingredients until combined well.

- Serve with warm tortillas or whole wheat chips.

Creamy Squash Soup

Ingredients

- acorn squash, cut lenthwise, seeds removed

- sweet potato, cut lenghtwise

- 4 shallots, cut lengthwise

- Tablespoons olive oil

- garlic cloves, whole

- Cups vegetable broth

- 14 Ounces cannellini beans, drained and rinsed

- 1/4 Cup sour cream

Instructions

- Preheat oven to 375 degrees.

- Brush cut sides of squash, sweet potato and shallots with oil. Place vegetables, cut side down, in a shallow roasting pan and add garlic cloves. Roast in oven until tender, about 30 – 40 minutes.

103

• Allow vegetables to cool, and scoop out flesh of squash, sweet potato. In a soup pot, place flesh of roasted vegetables, shallots and garlic.

• Add broth and bring to a boil. Reduce heat, and simmer, covered for 30 minutes, stirring occasionally.

• Pour half of the beans into the soup pot and allow soup to cool. Puree soup with a hand blender, until smooth.

• Add other half of beans and cream. Season to taste and simmer until warmed through, about 5 minutes. Serve.

Kidney Bean Soup

Ingredients

• 3 slices bacon

• 1 Teaspoon garlic cloves, minced

• 2 shallots, chopped

• carrots, chopped

• 28 Ounces kidney beans, drained

• 1/2 Cup quick cooking brown rice

• 4 Cups beef broth

• bay leaves

• 1/4 Teaspoon dried basil

Instructions

• In a large soup pot, cook bacon over medium heat until crisp. Crumble and set aside.

• In the same pan with the bacon oil, cook garlic, shallots and carrots until tender, about 5 minutes.

• Place the beans in blender and puree until smooth. Stir into the vegetable mixture in the pan.

• Add the bacon, rice, broth, bay leaves and basil. Stir soup and bring pot to a boil.

• Reduce heat and simmer covered, until rice is tender, 20 minutes. Serve.

Lentil Soup

Ingredients

• 2 Tablespoons olive oil

• onion, chopped

• carrots, chopped

• celery stalks, chopped

• medium potatoes, unpeeled, and cubed

• 2 bay leaf

- 2 Cups lentils, uncooked and rinsed

- 1/2 Teaspoon thyme

- 1/2 Teaspoon oregano

- Cups vegetable broth

- 3 Cups water

Instructions

- In a large soup pot, heat olive oil over medium- high heat.

- Add onion, carrots, celery, and potatoes. Cook for 7-8 minutes or until tender.

- Add bay leaves, lentils, thyme and oregano. Cook for a few more minutes.

- Add vegetable broth and water, bring to a boil. Reduce heat to low and let simmer, covered for another 45 minutes, until lentils are soft and fall apart.

Mushroom and Ginger Soup

Ingredients

- 2 Teaspoons vegetable oil

- 3 garlic cloves, crushed

- 1 Tablespoon fresh ginger, grated

- 4 Ounces white mushrooms, sliced

- 4 Cups vegetable broth

- 1 Teaspoon low sodium soy sauce

- 4 Ounces bean sprouts

- 4 Ounces whole wheat thin pasta

- 4 Tablespoons fresh cilantro

Instructions

- Bring a large pot of salted water to a boil. Add pasta and cook according to package instructions until al dente. Drain.

- In a large soup pot, heat oil over medium-high heat. Add garlic, ginger and mushrooms. Stir until softened, about 3-4 minutes.

- Add vegetable stock and bring to boil. Add soy sauce and bean sprouts and continue to cook until tender.

- To serve, place cooked noodles in individual bowls and ladle soup on top. Garnish with fresh cilantro

Mushroom Barley Soup

Ingredients

- 2 Tablespoons olive oil

* 1 Cup carrots, chopped

* 1 Cup onion, chopped

* 1 Pound white mushrooms, sliced

* 1 1/2 Cup smoked ham, chopped

* 28 Ounces chicken broth

* 14 Ounces stewed tomatoes, seedless

* 1/2 Cup quick cooking barley

Instructions

* In a large soup pot, heat olive oil over medium-high heat.

* Cook carrots and onion, stirring occasionally for about 5 minutes. Add mushrooms and cook, stirring frequently until mushrooms are tender, about 5 minutes.

* Add ham and cook stirring constantly for 1-2 minutes. Stir in chicken broth, tomatoes and barley.

* Bring pot to a boil, then reduce heat and simmer covered, until barley is tender, about 20 minutes.

Pea and Pesto Soup
Ingredients

* 1 Cup yellow split peas, uncooked, rinsed

- 2 Cups chicken broth

- 2 1/2 Cups water

- 2 Tablespoons pesto, homemade or store bought

- small zucchini, seeded and sliced

- 1/2 Cup green onions, chopped

Instructions

- In a large soup pot, combine split peas, broth and water and bring to a boil.

- Reduce heat, cover, and simmer for 20 minutes.

- Stir in pesto, zucchini, and green onions; simmer for 15 to 20 more minutes. Garnish with Parmesan cheese, if desired.

Asparagus Soup

Ingredients

- 1 Tablespoon olive oil

- 1 Cup shallots, finely chopped

- 3 garlic cloves, minced

- 2 Pounds asparagus, chopped into one inch pieces

- 6 Cups vegetable stock

• 1 Teaspoon salt

Instructions

• Reserve asparagus tops for later use. In a large soup pot, heat olive oil over medium heat. Cook shallots and garlic until softened, about 3-5 minutes.

• Add asparagus stalks, vegetable stock and salt and bring to a boil. Cover and reduce heat to low and simmer until asparagus softens.

• Let soup cool and puree with a hand blender, until creamy. Add asparagus tops and cook on medium for 5 minutes, until tops are tender.

Oatmeal Chocolate Chip Cookies

Ingredients

• 1/3 Cup brown sugar

• 1/2 Cup butter, softened

• 1/2 Teaspoon vanilla extract

• egg

• 1 Cup whole grain, rolled oats

• 3/4 Cups whole wheat flour

• 1/2 Teaspoon baking soda

• 1/2 Cup dark chocolate chips

Instructions

• Heat oven to 350 degrees. In a large bowl, cream brown sugar and butter until well combined. Stir in vanilla and egg and mix until light and fluffy. Stir in rolled oats, whole wheat flour, baking soda and fold in chocolate chips. Onto a cookie sheet covered with a Silpat mat or foil, drop the dough by rounded tablespoons (you can also use an ice cream scooper) about 2 inches apart.

• Bake 10-12 minutes or until golden brown. Cool slightly; remove from cookie sheet to a wire rack.

White Bean Puree

Ingredients

• 14 Ounces cannellini beans, drained and rinsed

• 2 garlic cloves

• 1/4 Cup fresh Italian parsley

• 1/2 lemon, juiced

• 1/4 Teaspoon oregano

• 1/2 Teaspoon salt

• 1/3 Cup olive oil

Instructions

• Blend all ingredients in a food processor until almost smooth. Serve with crusty bread, whole wheat crackers, or fresh vegetables

Baked Sweet Potato Fries

Ingredients

• 4 small sweet potatoes, unpeeled

• 1 Tablespoon butter, melted

• 1/4 Teaspoon salt

• dash of nutmeg

Instructions

• Preheat oven to 450F degrees. Spray a large baking pan with non-stick cooking spray.

• Scrub potatoes and cut lengthwise into quarters, then cut each quarter into 2 wedges. Arrange potatoes in a single layer in pan. In a small bowl, combine butter, salt, and nutmeg.

• Brush mixture onto potatoes and coat evenly. Bake in oven 20 minutes or until brown and tender.

Citrus Carrots

Ingredients

- 1 Pound baby carrots

- 2 Tablespoons balsamic vinegar

- 1/2 Cup orange juice

- orange, peeled and chopped

- 1 Tablespoon green onions, chopped finely

- 1 Tablespoon fresh dill, chopped

Instructions

- Steam carrots in a steamer until tender or plunge carrots into boiling water and cook for about 10 - 12 minutes until tender. Drain. Rinse with cold water and drain again.

- In a medium bowl, combine carrots, vinegar and orange juice. Stir to combine. Add orange segments, onions and dill. Lightly toss and serve.

Greek Lettuce Wraps

Ingredients

- 1/4 Cup mayonnaise

113

- 2 Teaspoons lemon juice

- 1/2 Cup white beans, drained and rinsed

- 1/3 Cup feta cheese,crumbled

- 2 Tablespoons pimentos, chopped

- 8 large lettuce leaves

- 1/2 Pound cooked chicken breast, cubed

Instructions

- In a medium bowl, combine mayonnaise and lemon juice.

- Stir in beans, mashing slightly with fork. Add cheese and pimentos, and mix lightly.

- Spread lettuce leaves evenly with bean mixture. Top with chicken; roll up. Serve.

Honey Baked Apples

Ingredients

- 4 apples, unpeeled

- 1/4 Cup brown sugar

- 1/2 Teaspoon ground cloves

- 1/2 Teaspoon cinnamon

- 1/2 Cup honey

- 1/2 Cup water

Instructions

- Preheat oven to 400 degrees.

- Core and slice apples into 1/2" rings. Place them in a shallow baking dish for later use.

- In a small saucepan, combine and heat brown sugar, cloves, cinnamon, honey and water.

- Pour over apples and bake 15 minutes or until tender, turning to baste once or twice. Serve.

CONCLUSION

The diverticulitis diet is a crucial component of managing this common gastrointestinal condition. By following a thoughtfully designed dietary plan, individuals with diverticulitis can find relief from acute symptoms, prevent future flare-ups, and maintain overall digestive health.

During an active diverticulitis episode, the primary goal is to give the digestive system a chance to rest and heal. This is accomplished through a liquid or low-fiber diet, which helps reduce inflammation and allow the inflamed pouches (diverticula) to recover. Clear broths, juices, and smooth, non-dairy-based soups are typically recommended during this acute phase.

As the inflammation subsides and the individual begins to feel better, the focus shifts to a high-fiber, plant-based diet. Whole grains, fresh fruits and vegetables, and legumes provide the necessary fiber to promote regular bowel movements and prevent further irritation. This gradual reintroduction of fiber-rich foods is crucial, as sudden increases can exacerbate symptoms.

Alongside the dietary changes, the diverticulitis diet also emphasizes the importance of staying hydrated, limiting foods that may cause gas or bloating, and avoiding red and processed meats, which can contribute to inflammation. Regular physical activity is also recommended, as it can help support healthy digestion.

It's important to remember that the diverticulitis diet is not a one-size-fits-all approach. Individual responses to certain foods and dietary components may vary, and it's essential to work closely with a healthcare provider to develop a personalized plan that takes into account your specific symptoms, dietary needs, and any other underlying medical conditions.

Through consistent adherence to the diverticulitis diet and other lifestyle modifications, many individuals are able to effectively manage their condition, reduce the risk of complications, and improve their overall quality of life. However, it's crucial to be patient and persistent when implementing dietary changes, as it may take time to find the right balance and to see the desired results.

In the long term, the diverticulitis diet aims to promote overall gut health and prevent future flare-ups. By providing the necessary nutrients, reducing inflammation, and supporting regular bowel movements, this dietary approach can help individuals with diverticulitis regain control over their digestive well-being.

In conclusion, the diverticulitis diet is a comprehensive and evidence-based approach to managing this common gastrointestinal condition. By following the dietary guidelines, individuals can find relief from acute symptoms, prevent future complications, and maintain a healthy digestive system. With the guidance of a healthcare provider and a commitment to the dietary changes, the diverticulitis diet can be a powerful tool in the management of this condition.